Calisthenics

Calisthenics for Beginner's: How to Make Your Dream Body

Bodyweight Exercises, Fitness, Workout Plan

Table of Contents

Introduction

If you want to live a long and healthy life, one of the things you should pay more attention to is physical fitness. When you do your best to be physically fit, part of a long and healthy life is being able to enjoy it through participation in your favorite activities and sports such as basketball, running or football among other activities. And when it comes to physical fitness, strength training is important.

But, in many cases, regular strength training requires a lot of equipment such as barbells, dumbbells and other resistance training machines or contraptions. A home gym requires significant investment and space while enrolling in a gym may also prove to be costly, especially if your budget's tight. If such is the case, is there a way for you to get enough significant strength or resistance training for optimal physical fitness? My answer is a resounding "YES!"

Calisthenics is a strength training method or technique that doesn't require barbells, dumbbells or other weight lifting equipment. All you need is your body and a couple of fixed items such as a pole, overhead bar in the park or playground, or a bench and you're good to go! And in this book, you will discover why you should get into calisthenics and, more importantly, how to perform callisthenic exercises in order to build up your strength and become and stay physically fit. And as you master the art of calisthenics, you'll also enjoy the freedom of being able to train your body for strength anytime and anywhere. You won't be a slave to the gym and its fancy but pricey equipment or membership fees.

Are you ready to learn how to get a fit and strong body using nothing else but the body you have now? If so, what are you waiting for? Turn the page and start reading!

Chapter 1: It's All about Your Body

As mentioned earlier, calisthenic exercises – a.k.a. calisthenics – is the term that is used to describe a set of resistance or strength-training exercises that don't use "artificial" weights like dumbbells, barbells and other weight-lifting machines but instead use a person's own bodyweight. Calisthenics doesn't just tone and strengthen your muscles but it also improves their endurance. And in case you're interested in the word's etymology, it comes from two Greek words "kalos" and "sthenos" that mean beauty and strength, respectively.

Often times, people think of calisthenics as resistance training for beginners only, i.e., it's not for building serious strength and fitness. Just because calisthenics is one of the most ideal types of resistance or strength training for beginners doesn't mean it's exclusive for them only. Even if you consider yourself to be relatively fit or have been doing strength training for quite a while now, you can still enjoy many benefits from incorporating calisthenics into your training regimen. But regardless if you're a beginner or someone who's got a bit of experience with strength or resistance training already, this book has you covered.

If you're a beginner, you may be wondering what benefits you can enjoy if you consider calisthenics as your primary strength and fitness training method?   One benefit is consistency or regularity of exercise. Why? It's because, as I mentioned earlier, calisthenics uses no special training equipment. You only need your body, which you can never really get away from unless you're practicing astral projection or worse, are already dead, and some common items that you can find practically anywhere such as a fixed and immovable object such as a pole, a door, an overhead bar, and a bench or sturdy chair. As such, you really won't have any excuses – other than you're sick, injured, or just plain lazy – for not being able to regularly workout.

The second benefit you may enjoy from doing calisthenics is improved mastery of your body. You may be thinking you're already the master of your body as you're able to make it do whatever you want to do, e.g., walk, run, jump, poo, pee, hold your poo, hold your pee and make really weird noises, among other things, and that all bases are practically covered when it comes to body mastery. Well, you're wrong! There are still areas of bodily control that you can significantly improve on such as proprioception (the capability to sense movements within your body's joints and joint positions), coordination, self-awareness, and balance.

If you're highly reliant on exercise machines such as Smith machines, lat pull-down machines, press machines and leg extension machines, among others, for your strength or resistance training, you train your body to move along a fixed line and range of motion that's naturally limited by the machine's range of motion. What this means is that when you're doing bench press using a machine for example, you can go all out without having to use other auxiliary muscles because the machine's fixed range of motion ensures perfect balance even if you don't use auxiliary muscles such as the shoulders, the stomach or core muscles and back muscles. Do this long enough and consistently enough and you'll eventually end up with less ability to balance because you leave out the development of other auxiliary muscles.

When it comes to athletic performance, you need optimum strength and balance to go hand in hand. You won't be able to shoot 3-point shots as quickly and accurately as Steph Curry if you're not able to achieve excellent balance for a quick jump shot after a quick stop-and-pop move. Even a sport that's not as strenuous as basketball such as golf, require a great sense of body balance to be able to hit a perfect swing. When you work with your body weight, you have no choice but to learn how to be aware of how you move your body to keep your body balanced as you execute calisthenic exercises. And such learned awareness and balance is key to optimal athletic performance.

And even if you're a person who's already doing strength and fitness training via weights, you can still benefit much from incorporating calisthenics into your routine. How? Aside from much improved balance, you can also develop agility and flexibility, which can help you perform much better in sports. Most of the time, serious weight lifters tend to be an inflexible bunch with limited ranges of motion, especially bodybuilders and power lifters.

If you want proof of such, consider specific groups of people whose strength and fitness-training routines are primarily based on calisthenics. One of them is the late great Muhammad Ali! If you ever get the chance to watch video clips of his fights and take a look at how most, if not all, heavyweight boxers move these days, you can see one startling difference: Ali literally flies like a butterfly and stings like a bee! And such combination of strength and agility cannot be replicated by barbells and dumbbells based training method. He's both strong and fast because most of his training is calisthenics-based. The GOAT's (greatest of all time) coach made him go through a program that was mostly based on bodyweight or calisthenic exercises because he believed that it was simply the best way for boxers to train.

Another popular and well-known testimony to the benefits of calisthenics is Jason Statham, best known for his roles in blockbuster movies like The Transporter series, Spy, and the last two "Fast and the Furious" movies. He's buffed, strong and agile. His secret? Calisthenics! Ever imagine how he's able to maintain such level of fitness, strength, and agility considering his very hectic schedule as an action star, which is mostly comprised of location shootings where gyms and gym equipment aren't part of the normal environment? Well, wonder no more because calisthenics, as mentioned earlier, can be performed practically anywhere.

Gerard Butler, a.k.a., King Leonidas of the hit movie 300 is another powerful testimony to calisthenics' benefits. He and the rest of the buffed and fit Spartans used calisthenics to supplement their strength building workouts in order to get ripped and muscular. You can use calisthenics too to train like a Spartan!

One of the world's most feared fighters is the Dragon himself, Bruce Lee. Most people see his speed, power and, of course, his ripped and shredded body in each and every movie he's ever done where he kicks the living hell out of all his opponents. And guess what, those are products of a strength and fitness method that's primarily grounded on calisthenics.

Lastly, consider real life badass warriors that are able to accomplish what most people deem to be impossible – special armed forces groups such as the Marines and the Navy SEALs. Most – if not all – of their exercises are calisthenics from burpees, to pushups and pull-ups, among many others. You hardly find gym time for these ultra-fit, strong, and agile men who fight battles that you only hear of in movies and novels. Their practically today's version of the Spartans. They rely primarily on calisthenics because they can't afford to bulk up too much like bodybuilders and power lifters because doing so will significantly limit their mobility, agility and flexibility. With such limited physical traits, they won't be able to do many critical mission-related things like carry a lot of gear, walk long distances carrying such and get out of tight spots.

Now that you know why you should do calisthenics, i.e., its benefits, it's time to get to the meat of this book and learn how to perform calisthenic exercises to help you get that dream body you desire!

Chapter 2: Basic Calisthenic Movements - Legs

When it comes to getting that dream body you've always dreamed off, it's important to be able to burn as many calories as possible. To do that, you must perform exercises that burn the most calories. Exercises that involve the biggest muscle groups help you burn the most calories and body fat.

The legs are your body's biggest group of muscles, which makes them the primary muscles to workout for optimal weight loss. And more than just burning as many calories as possible, your legs are crucial when it comes to performing many of your body's basic movements, from walking to standing up, to lifting stuff off the ground. As such, strong legs are a necessity.

Before we dive right into the best calisthenic exercises for your legs, let's talk about the specific muscles in the group. The first one is your thigh and its primary function is to extend or straighten your legs. Given this primary function, the best way to exercise your thighs for strength is to straighten your legs – from a bent position – against resistance or weight. Then you stand up or jump, you straighten your legs against resistance.

The second muscle of the group is your hamstring, which is the big muscle directly beneath your buttock muscle and behind your thigh. If the thigh's function is to straighten your leg, the hamstring's function is the opposite – to curl or bend your leg. The best way to strengthen your hamstring muscles is to bend your legs at the knee – as if trying to let your heels touch your buttocks – against some type of resistance.

The final part of your leg muscle group is the calf. The primary function of the calf is to elevate or push your body upward using your foot. If you want to exercise your calf muscles, the best way to do it is to push your body upward against resistance using your foot, i.e., tiptoeing.

Now that you know the individual functions of the muscles comprising your legs, let's proceed with leg calisthenics.

Squats

When you perform squatting exercises, you work out the upper leg muscles, which are your hamstrings and thighs. You also work out auxiliary muscles such as your calf, lower back and abdominal muscles because those muscles help you balance your body as you perform the exercise. Because they work out 2 of your body's biggest muscles as well as several other muscles, squats are probably the best exercise for burning calories and body fat.

Here's how to perform squats:

- Assume the starting position by standing straight with both feet about shoulder-width apart. Place both your hands either at the sides of your head or behind it.

- Gradually lower your body – keeping your lower back straight – until you're assuming a squatting position. While doing this, always keep your lower back straight, eyes focused forward, and both your feet securely planted on the ground.

- When your thighs and hamstrings are already parallel to the floor, that's your cue that you're already at an optimal squatting position. Hold the position for at least 2 seconds before lifting your body back up until you're back at the starting position. This constitutes 1 complete repetition or rep. Perform 3 sets of 10 to 20 reps each per workout.

In order to minimize your risks for injuries, always remember to keep your lower back straight all throughout the movement. You must also be conscious of not letting your knees extend past your toes as you squat. Imagine there's a vertical line extending from the tips of your toes. Make sure your toes never breach that line because, if they do, you subject your knees to excessive strain that may lead to pain or injury in the long run.

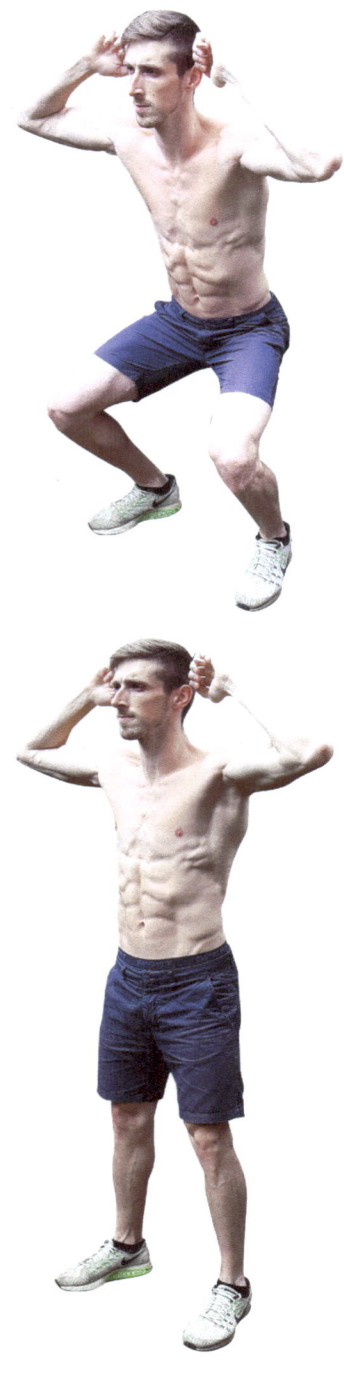

Leg Curls

This is your primary exercise for working out your hamstring muscles. Here's how to perform it:

- Assume the starting position by standing straight beside a doorpost or in front of a wall. Place one hand on the doorpost or wall to balance yourself as you perform the exercise.

- Start by bending your right leg as if you're trying to touch your buttocks with your right heel while keeping your right thigh straight or perpendicular to the ground all throughout the movement. At the top of the movement, pause and hold the position for a second or two before bringing back to starting position. Do 10 to 20 reps before doing the same with your left leg. Do 3 sets of 10 to 20 reps for each leg.

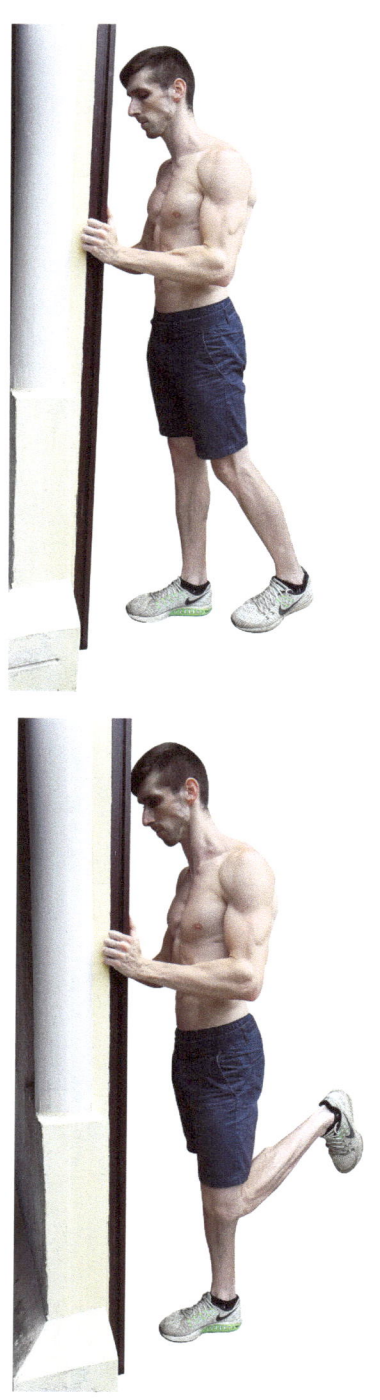

Lunges

After working out your thighs and hamstrings, it's time to workout your thighs again but this time together with your butt muscles. To perform lunges:

- Assume the starting position by stepping forward with your right leg while keeping your left foot planted on the ground by the balls and toes right behind you. Your left foot's heel should be lifted at this point while your whole right foot is planted on the ground in front of you.

- With your eyes fixed ahead and your lower back straight, start bringing down your body in a lunging motion, keeping your right foot and your left foot's ball and toes firmly planted on the ground. While doing this, both your knees will bend. Stop short of your left knee kissing the ground and hold the position for a second or two before bringing your body back up to the starting position. Do 10 to 20 reps before switching legs (step forward with the left foot and your right foot behind) to do the same. Do 3 sets of 10 to 20 reps for each leg.

- Always be mindful of keeping your lower back straight all throughout the movement and make sure that the knee of your forward stepping leg doesn't go past the toe line, as is the case with squats, in order to minimize risks for lower back and knee injuries, respectively.

This particular exercise is crucial if you want to gain the necessary leg and knee strength, which are both needed for performing athletic movements that require sudden bursts of speed (sprinting, ankle-breaking basketball moves ala-Kyrie Irving and Steph Curry), jumping high when executing volleyball spikes or dunking the basketball high above the rim, or executing long running jumps as in the case of, well, long jumps.

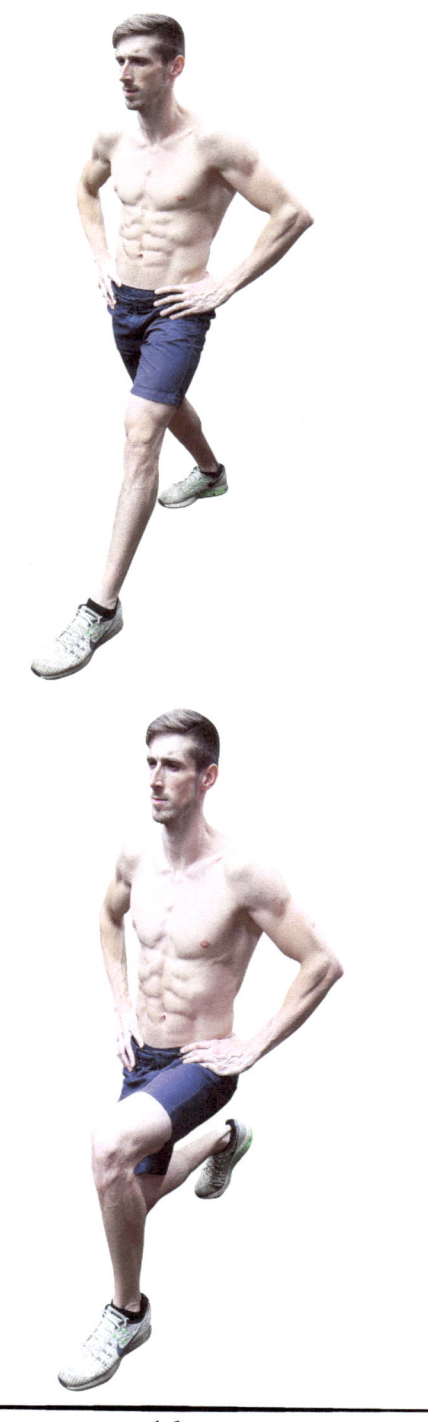

Calf Raises

As the exercise's name implies, this one's for strengthening your calf muscles, which are crucial for activities that require jumping and running. Strong calf muscles also provide you with the ability to eke out those final pushes such as the case with jumping high or sprinting. And here's how you do this exercise:

- Assume the starting position by standing on the edge of an elevated surface such as a stair step or a sturdy box or platform, with only the ball and toes of your right foot. Hold on to a wall, post, rail or something that's sturdy and fixed for assistance in keeping balanced.

- Lower your body slowly and after going as low as you can, lift your body up as high as you can using only your right foot and right calf muscle. Hold the position for a second or two before descending all the way down again. Do 10 to 20 reps before switching to the left calf muscle and performing 10 to 20 reps as well. Perform 3 sets of 10 to 20 reps per leg.

- Always keep your lower back straight. Use your hand simply to give you that extra "balance", putting the primary burden of balancing yourself on the leg you're working out to improve your overall balance.

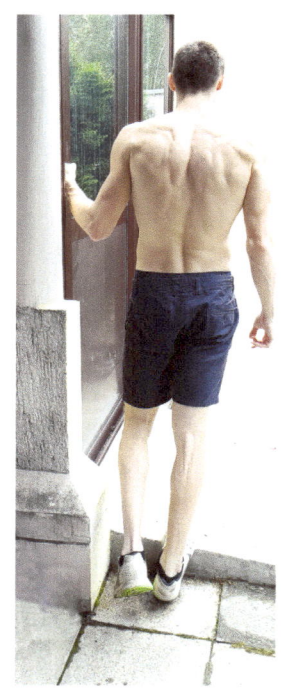

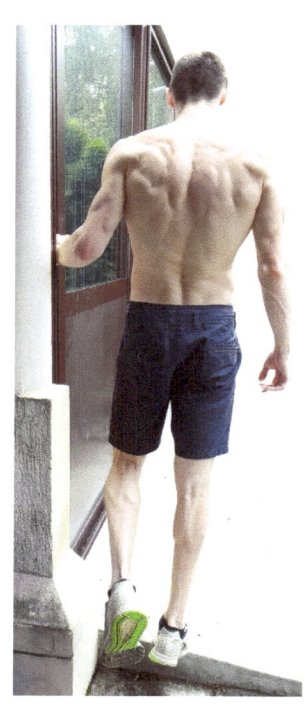

Chapter 3: Basic Calisthenic Movements - Back

The next largest muscle group in your body is in your back, which means exercising it helps burn a lot of calories and body fat too. This is a very important muscle group to strengthen but most people ignore or take this group for granted, resulting in chronic pain or worse, injuries. It's probably because the back isn't as "sexy" as other muscles like the chest, abs, shoulders, and arms.

Fortunately, most back pains can be addressed by performing simple back-strengthening exercises. That's why more than just burning more calories and fat, you should regularly exercise your back to minimize your risks for one of the most common kinds of pain and injury. And in this chapter, you'll learn some of the best calisthenic exercises for your back.

Pull Ups

This exercise will strengthen both your middle and upper back muscles and to perform this, you'll need a very sturdy overhead bar that's high enough to let your feet stay above ground from a hanging position, such as the kinds you see on parks, playgrounds, or even at home. Here's how you do it:

- Jump and hang on to an overhead bar with your palms facing forward, i.e., an overhand grip. Allow yourself to hang from the bar for a second or two before beginning the exercise.

- Pull yourself up the bar until your chest touches the bar. If you aren't strong enough yet, pull yourself up as far as you can. Count to two before lowering your body back to the original hanging position in a controlled manner.

- Perform the movement for 10 to 20 repetitions for the first set. Rest for at most 1 minute before doing 2 more sets of 10 to 20 repetitions.

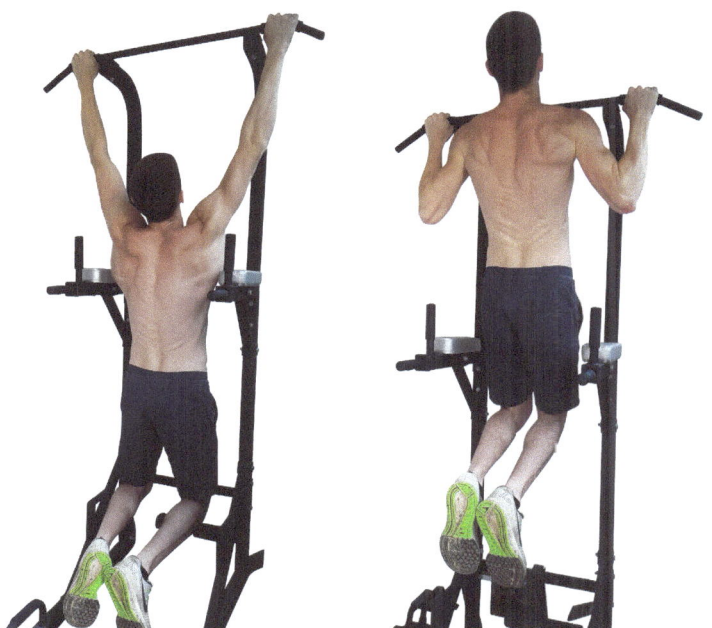

Keep in mind that for most beginners, bodyweight is too heavy a weight to correctly work with from top to bottom with the prescribed number of reps. If you're not able to perform the regular version just yet, you can do the light version of this exercise instead:

- Jump as high as you can so that you start from a position where your chest is as close to the overhead bar as possible, still using an overhand grip. Start pulling from that position if your chest has neither touched the bar yet nor is near to doing so and hold the position at the top of the movement for a count of two before gradually bringing your body down to a hanging position. But if your chest already touches or is close to touching the bar, just hold the position for a count of two before lowering down your body to a completely hanging position.

- Let go of the bar so you can go back to the ground and jump again as high as you can to repeat the movement 9 to 19 times more for a total of 10 to 20 reps. Perform 3 sets of the exercise.

When you're strong enough, transition to the standard version of the pull-ups.

Chin Ups

This exercise also strengthens your middle and upper back muscles and as with the pull-ups, you'll need an overhead bar that's high enough to let you hang completely with your feet off the ground. The only difference is the grip. Here, your palms will be facing towards you, i.e., an underhand grip, at shoulder width. To perform this exercise's standard version:

- Jump so you can grab the overhead bar with an underhand grip, letting your body hang for a second or two before executing the movement.

- Start pulling your body up to the point that your chin is able to make contact with the bar. At the top of the movement, hold your position for a count of two before lowering yourself down in a controlled manner until completely hanging, which constitutes one repetition or rep. Perform 3 sets of 10 to 20 repetitions per set.

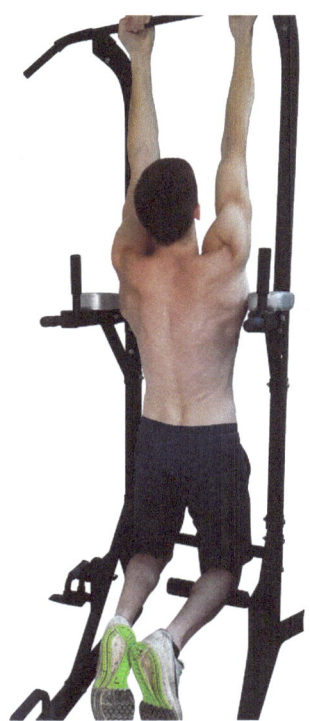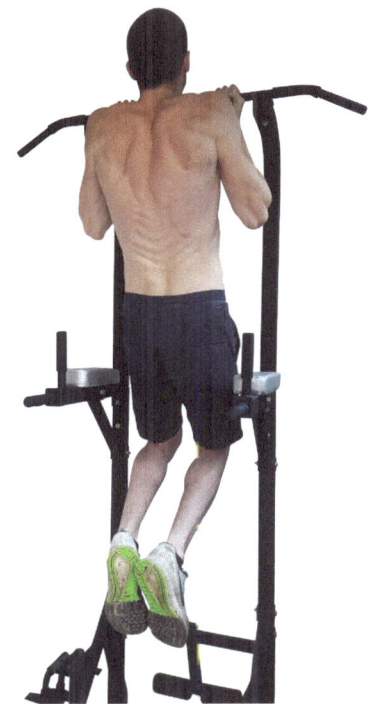

And just like the pull ups, the chin ups also has a beginner's version or a "light" version, which you can perform simply by jumping as high as you can so you either start pulling yourself up from a much higher position or touch the bar with your chin already. Either way, hold your position at the top of the movement, i.e., chin touching the bar, for a count of two before lowering yourself down gradually to a hanging position before letting go and coming back down to the ground. That's one repetition. Perform 3 sets of 10 to 20 repetitions each.

Super Man

This exercise focuses mainly on strengthening your lower back. Here's how you can act like Clark Kent in strengthening your precious lower back muscles:

- Lie flat on a mat facing down with your arms fully extended upwards, as if you're preparing to fly upward like Super Man.

- To perform 1 repetition, raise both your arms and thighs off the floor, hold for a count of two, and lower them to return to your starting position. As a beginner, do only as many as you can. But over time, you'll need to build up to doing 10 to 20 reps per set and perform 3 sets per workout.

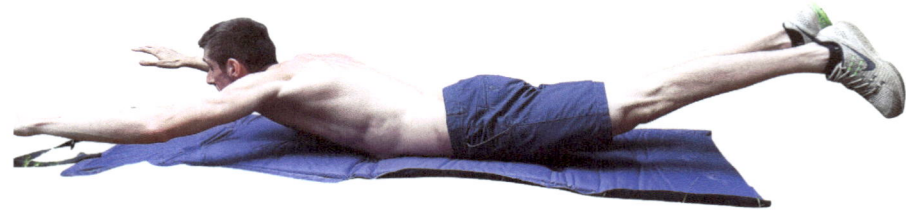

Hand Ups

As with the Super Man, this exercise helps strengthen your lower back muscles. Here's how to perform this exercise:

- Assume the same starting position as the Super Man, i.e., lie down on a mat face down with your arms stretched upward as if you're about to fly off the ground.

- Press the floor with your toes and, while doing so, try to lift your hands and arms as high above the floor as you possibly can, with your arms and back staying straight all throughout the movement.

- After reaching the top of the movement, bring your hands and arms back down to the starting position. This is one repetition. Build up to doing 3 sets of 10 to 20 repetitions each per workout.

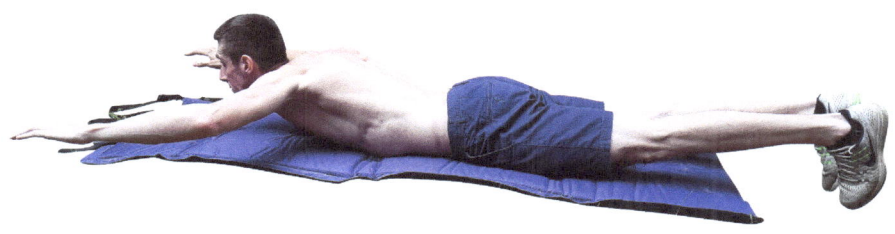

Toe Ups

This final exercise also works your lower back muscles and is the opposite of the hand up. To do this:

- Start by lying on a mat face down, with your arms stretched up as far above your head as possible, as if you're about to fly.

- This time, press your hands firmly on the floor and, as you do, lift your thighs as high as possible off the floor before bringing them back down. This constitutes one repetition. Gradually build up to doing 3 sets of 10 to 20 reps each per workout.

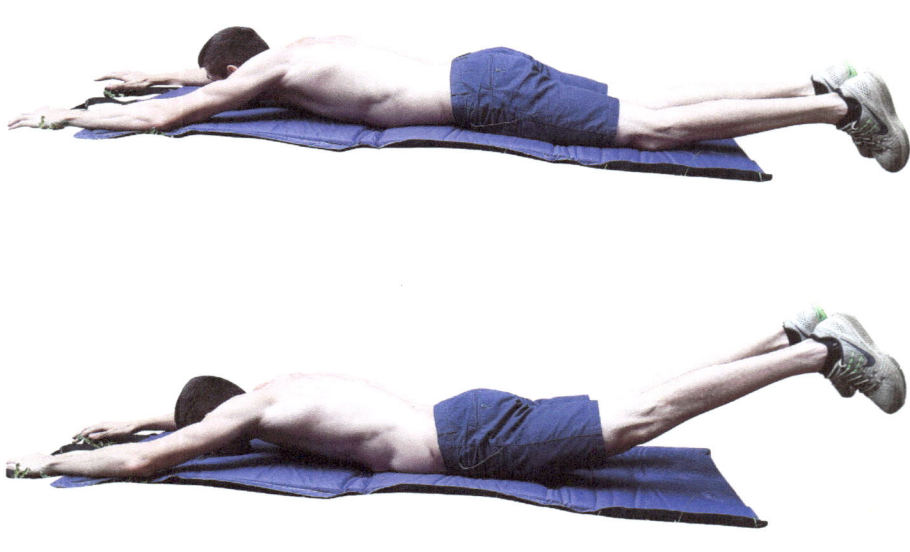

Chapter 4: Basic Calisthenic Movements - Core

Many people train their core muscles primarily for vanity's sake, i.e., they want to have shredded and ripped six-pack abs to show off at the beach or just about anywhere else it's completely legal to walk around shirtless. But there is an even bigger and more important benefit to performing core exercises, which is to strengthen your core muscles. These are crucial if you want to be able to minimize your risks for injuries while improving athletic performance, e.g., moving faster and becoming stronger. And in this chapter, we'll focus on exercises that can help you not just to have a toned or ripped set of abs but have strong core muscles.

Crunches

Crunches help you develop abdominal muscle strength in your upper abs. To perform them:

- Assume the starting position by lying on a mat flat on your back. For your feet you have 3 options: rest them on an elevated surface like a bench or chair so that your thighs stay perpendicular to the floor, lift your legs up so that your thighs are perpendicular to the floor, or plant your feet on the floor as close as possible to your buttock muscles. However, the optimal position for me is the one where you lift your legs up without any support, which will train you to balance your body as well.

- With your hands in a crossed position on your chest, start lifting your chest up as high as possible, as if attempting to touch your knees with them. At the topmost part of the movement, squeeze and hold your abdominal muscles for a count of two before lowering your chest down to starting position in a controlled manner. This is one repetition. Perform 3 sets of 10 to 20 reps per set.

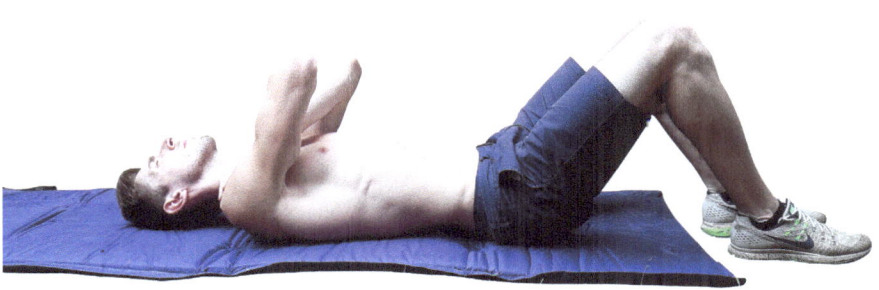

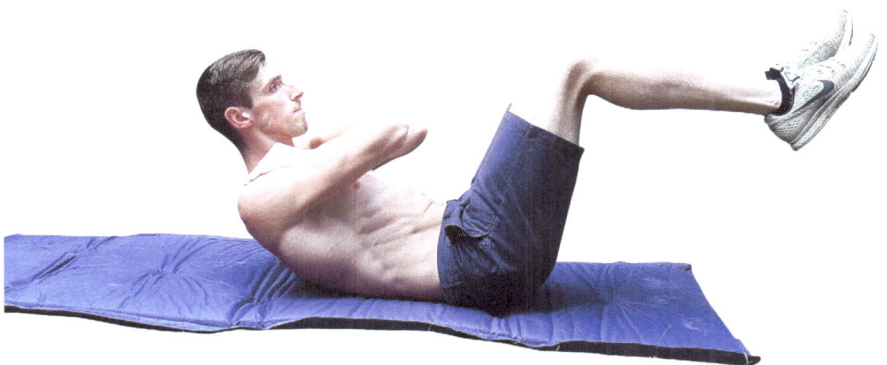

All throughout the movement, always keep your lower back planted on the ground to maximize the effort and minimize your risk for lower back injuries.

Reverse Crunches

If crunches help you strengthen your upper abs, then reverse crunches strengthen the lower one. To do this correctly:

- Assume the starting position by lying flat on your back on a mat.

- Bend your knees so that they form a 90-degree angle while still keeping your feet on the ground.

- Press your hands on the floor, at the level of your buttocks and lift your feet off the ground – keeping the 90-degree angle all throughout the movement – by rocking your pelvis. Bring your knees as close as you possibly can to your chest.

- Hold and squeeze your abdominal muscles at the top of the movement for a count of two before bringing your feet down to the starting position. This is one repetition. Gradually build up to doing 3 sets of 10 to 20 reps per set.

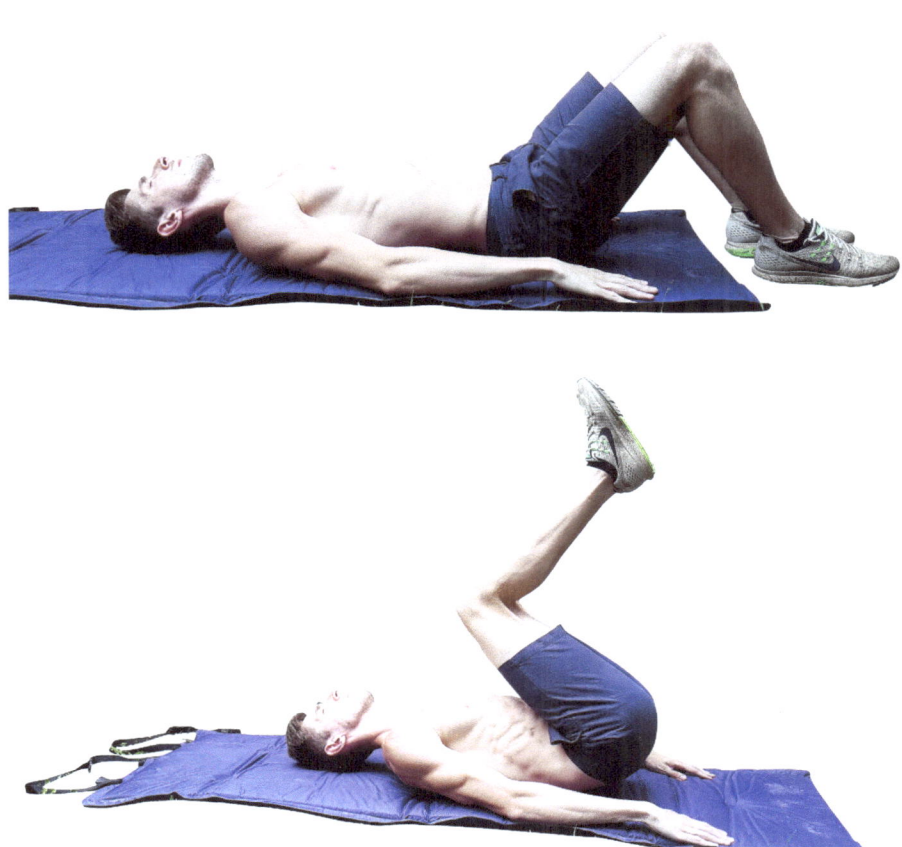

After your abdominal muscles have already grown accustomed to this exercise and you're able to easily finish 3 sets of up to 20 reps each, you can increase the intensity by widening the angle of your knees, i.e., extending your feet and legs. The straighter your legs are, the harder it becomes to perform the repetitions.

Planks

This is an exercise that strengthens both your abs and lower back muscles – your complete core group of muscles. To perform this:

- Start by lying on a mat face down.

- Lift your upper body by bracing both your elbows on the floor just around the chest or nipple area.

- Lift the rest of our body by bracing your lower body with your toes, forming a straight line or plank. At this point, only your elbows and toes should be touching the ground.

- Hold this position for 30 seconds or if you can't just yet, gradually build up to 30 seconds. Return to the starting position, which is one repetition. Gradually build up to doing 3 sets of 10 to 20 reps each.

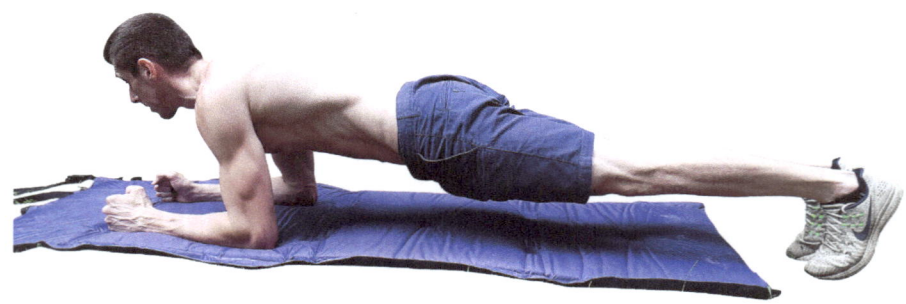

Butt Lifts

No, this isn't some sort of plastic surgery procedure. This is a core strengthening exercise that helps you strengthen your lower back, abdominal and butt muscles in one fell swoop! To do this:

- Start by assuming the same position for beginning the reverse crunch, which is lying on a mat on your back, knees bent at a 90-degree angle, and both your feet firmly planted on the ground.

- With you hands pressed on the floor at the sides, bring your buttocks off the floor as high as you possibly can, hold the position for a count of two, then bring your buttocks back down to the floor in a controlled manner. That's one repetition. Gradually build up to doing 3 sets of 10 to 20 reps each.

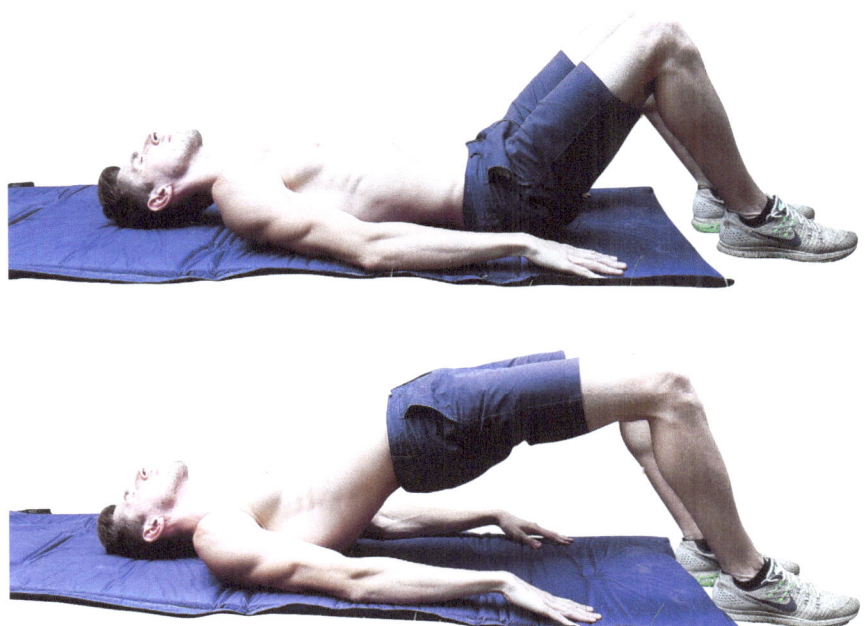

While performing this exercise, always keep your lower back straight. Doing so will not only help you optimally perform the exercise but also help you to minimize risks of lower back injury.

Chapter 5: Basic Calisthenic Movements - Chest

The chest is one of the best body parts to showcase when it comes to attracting other people, whether as a man or a woman. Big chests look good on either male or female but when it comes to men, bigger means more muscular. And of all muscles, the chest is the one most related to physical strength. Proof of this is how most men tend to brag about how strong they are in lifting, which is by bragging about how heavy they're able to bench press at the gym.

In this chapter, I'll show you some of the best calisthenic exercises that don't just build strong chests but also flexible ones.

Push Ups

Oh yeah, this one's a no-brainer. But even if it's a given when it comes to developing a stronger and bigger chest, many people aren't able to do so because they do it wrong. Here's how to do it right:

- Assume the starting position of a plank exercise. In this case, however, you'll be using your hands and fully extended arms to lift your upper body instead of your elbows. Your hands must be about slightly wider than shoulder width and at chest level area. Your lower body's still lifted up by your toes and your body should stay straight all throughout the exercise.

- Lower your body with your chest close to touching the ground, which will be the movement's starting point. Push your upper body off the ground with your arms, pivoting at the toes while keeping your whole body straight.

- Stop short of fully extending your arms, i.e., short of locking out your elbows, hold the position for 2 seconds, then bring our body back down with your chest close to touching the ground. This is one repetition. Build up to 3 sets of 10 to 20 reps each.

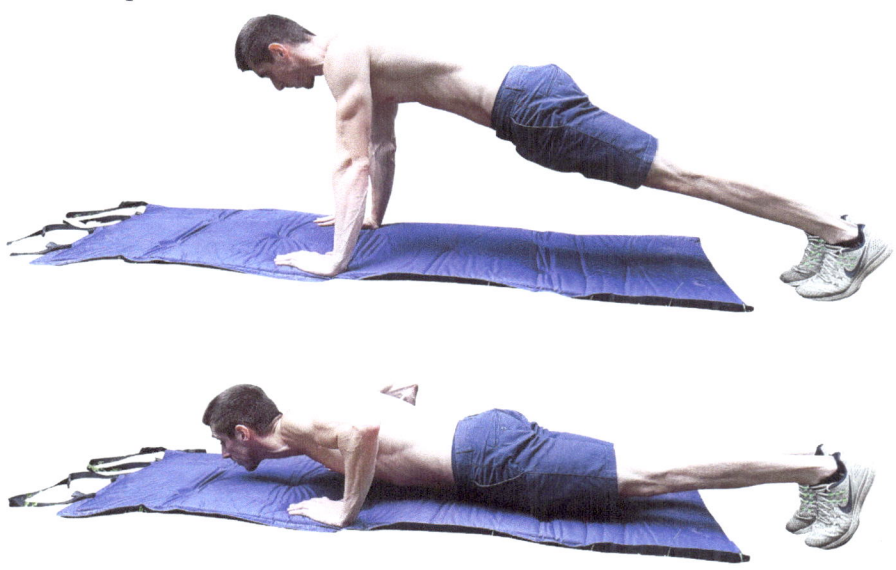

To optimally work out your chest muscles, let it carry the load instead of sharing it with your shoulder muscles. How can you do this? Keep your shoulders pulled back all throughout the movement to isolate the chest and ensure that it bears the brunt of the load.

To minimize your risk of injuring your elbows, stop short of locking out at the top of the movement. Why? When you lock your elbows out, you inadvertently make your elbows bear all your body weight. By stopping short of locking out, you keep all the weight on the chest and triceps instead of your elbow joints, thereby reducing your risks for injuring your elbows.

Counter Top Push Ups

For most people, push-ups can be a very challenging exercise to perform. As a beginner, you might need to start with a lighter version of the standard pushups. One of them is the counter top push-ups. And here's how you can do it:

- Assume the starting position of a regular pushup. This time however, you'll be placing your hands on the edge of a fixed kitchen counter top or a very sturdy and steady table.

- With your hands at slightly wider than shoulder width positions on the edge of a kitchen or table top and your arms fully extended, take several steps backward so that you're in a typical starting position for performing pushups, only that your hands aren't on the floor but on the edge of a tabletop. Keep your body straight and your shoulders drawn back at all times.

- Lower your chest to touch or almost touching the edge of the kitchen top or table to begin the movement.

- Push your body up until your arms stop short of locking out. Hold the position for a count of two before bringing your upper body back down to the edge of the kitchen or tabletop. This is one repetition. Do 3 sets of 10 to 20 repetitions each.

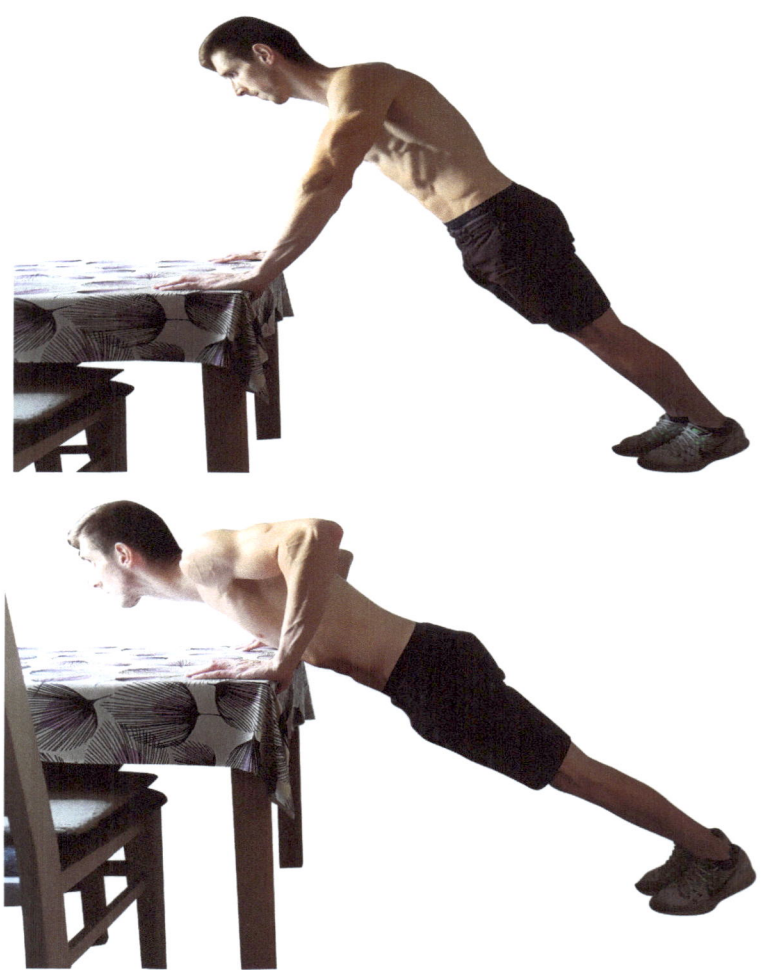

As with the regular push ups, always keep your body straight, don't lock your elbows, and keep your shoulders drawn back to maximize and isolate the weight on the chest and minimize risk for injuries.

Praying Push Ups

Well, it's actually called kneeling push ups. But since kneeling is always associated with praying, I took the liberty of modifying the name. Or you can also call it the begging-for-mercy push-ups, as kneeling is associated with such too. Anyway, this is as beginner's level as you can get with push-ups. It's like if you can't perform 3 sets of 10 to 20 reps each, there might not be hope for you anymore! But seriously speaking, this is as basic and easy as any push ups can get that's why I'm confident that even with a weak set of chest muscles, you can perform push ups and build up towards performing regular push ups for 3 sets of 10 to 20 reps each.

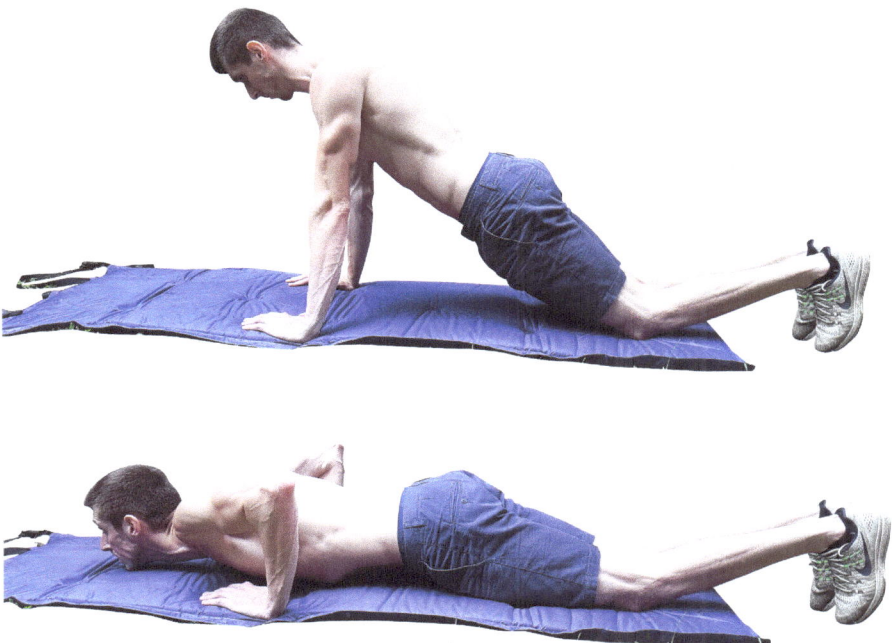

Performing this is simple and easy. Just kneel on all fours and perform 3 sets of 20 pushups each. It's that easy!

Chapter 6: Basic Calisthenic Movements - Shoulders

Next to the chest, shoulders are another strong way to look strong and sexy. Broad shoulders make men look really macho and sexy and relatively wide shoulders help emphasize women's tiny waists – oolalah! But more than just a weapon of mass vanity, strong shoulders help you easily perform movements that require lifting and overhead throwing such as shooting jump shots (basketball), throwing shot puts and javelins, and clean jerks. Even if you're not an athlete, strong shoulders help you move heavier weights with ease and safety over your head, such as when putting heavy things on your overhead cupboards or cabinets. And in this chapter, I'll show you some of the best flexibility and strength and muscle building calisthenic exercises for shoulders.

Shoulder Circles

Doing this regularly helps you improve and maintain excellent flexibility in your shoulders. You can do this by standing straight with your legs slightly separated for a relatively stable but comfortable base. Then, move our arms in a circular motion, starting by bringing them forward then rotating them backwards in a circular motion before rotating them back to the original position by reversing the movement. That's one repetition. Perform 3 sets of at least 20 repetitions each.

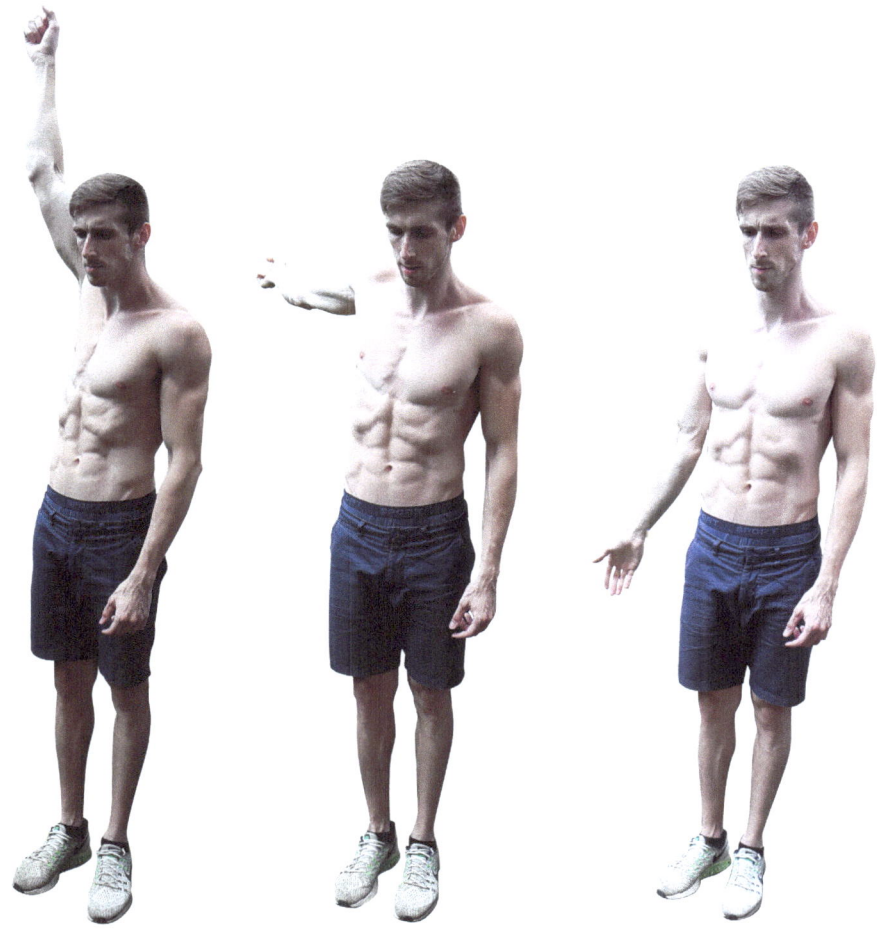

Rolling Planks

This particular movement allows you to strengthen and build your shoulder's side muscles, which are called side deltoids or side delts. To do the rolling planks:

- Start by doing a plank, i.e., your body straight with only your elbows and toes touching the ground.

- From this position, roll to your right side first by resting your full body weight on your right elbow and your toes still planted on the ground while keeping your body as straight as an arrow.

- Move your left arm as far back as possible, keeping it straight at all times. Hold the stretch for two seconds before going back to your original planking position and rolling to the left side, this time by resting your weight on the left elbow and pulling your straight right arm as far back as possible before going back to the original planking position. That's one repetition. Build up to doing 3 sets of 10 to 20 repetitions each.

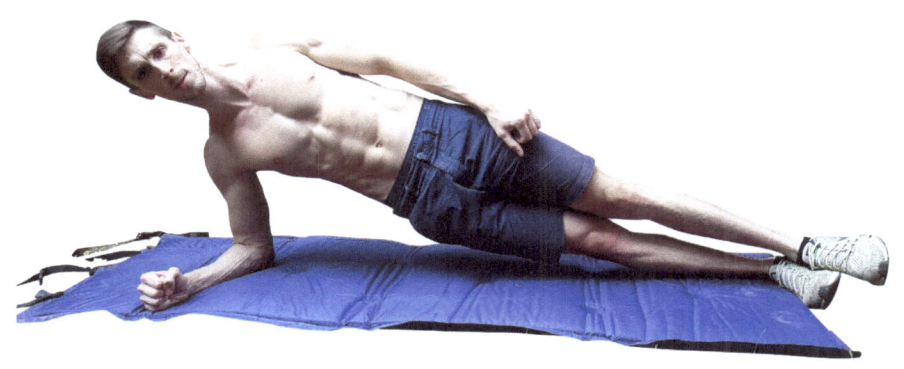

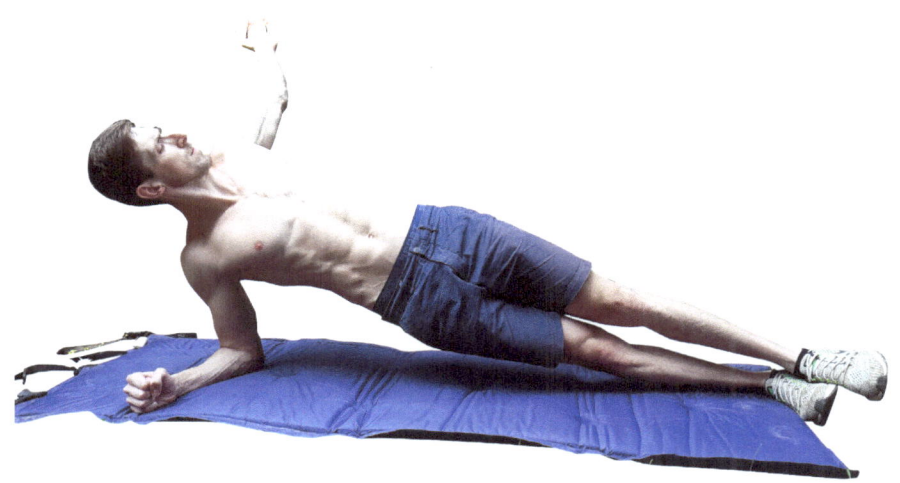

Chapter 7: How It All Looks Together

Now that you've learned the best basic calisthenic or bodyweight exercises for each of your body's major muscle groups, it's about time for you to see how they all fit together to help you achieve and keep your dream body. These exercises are by no means an exhaustive list but by giving you the basic movements, I've given you the basic foundations from which you can add to your basic starting calisthenics routine later on.

By giving you a basic idea for a routine, you'll be able to learn how to create your own later on. And as you do, you'll be able to achieve complete independence in terms of calisthenics and be able to consistently workout anytime and anywhere. Nothing will hold you back from regularly performing strength exercises en route to creating that dream body you've always desired and keep it.

Your ideal calisthenics routine is a full-body workout. This means – as you can glean from the term – that you will be exercising all your major muscle groups in one workout session. This means every time you work out, you'll be training your legs, back, core, chest, and shoulder muscles. Don't worry about the arms because by working out your chest and back, you'll inadvertently be working out your triceps and biceps, respectively.

Always keep in mind that building strength, muscle mass, and flexibility shouldn't be your top priority when working out. It should be safety. As such, I'd like you to keep a couple of things in mind. First, always perform the exercises using proper form. If you find you're only able to perform 5 reps with proper form as compared to 10 with a sloppy one, go for 5 reps.

The second thing I want you to always keep in mind is that as a beginner, don't expect yourself to be able to perform all the exercises completely, i.e., 3 sets of up to 20 reps each. If you find yourself physically unable to complete the prescribed sets and reps, no need to beat yourself up about it. Just do as much as you can and build up towards the prescribed sets and reps.

Ok, now that I've got those two things off my chest, allow me to give you a sample routine that you can start working with as a beginner. As you reach the point of comfort when performing all the exercises with the prescribed number of sets and reps, you can modify the routines to include more exercises or replace them with more challenging ones.

For the first month as a beginner, you may want to start with this routine building up from your best efforts to the following prescribed reps and sets:

- Legs: Squats 10 to 12 reps for 2 sets.

- Back: Toe Ups. 10 to 12 reps for 2 sets.

- Core: Planks 10 to 12 reps for 2 sets.

- Core: Butt Lifts 10 to 12 reps for 2 sets.

- Chest: Praying Push Ups: 10 to 12 reps for 2 sets.

- Shoulders: Rolling Planks 10 to 12 reps for 2 sets.

When you're able to do them consistently, you can now increase the intensity of your workouts by adapting this routine:

- Squats: Squats 10 to 20 reps for 3 sets.

- Legs: Lunges 10 to 20 reps for 3 sets per leg.

- Back: Toe Ups. 10 to 20 reps for 3 sets.

- Core: Planks 10 to 20 reps for 3 sets.

- Core: Butt Lifts 10 to 20 reps for 3 sets.

- Chest: Counter Top Push Ups 10 to 20 reps for 3 sets.

- Shoulders: Shoulder rounds as many as possible.

Have you now got a sense of how it all looks from the sample routine above? Remember, it's crucial that you're able to perform at least one exercise for each major muscle group and progressively build up towards the prescribed 3 sets of 10 to 20 reps each for all exercises. And more importantly, make sure you get enough rest and recuperation – 48 hours – in between workouts. In other words, wait for at least 2 days from the time you last worked out before working out again. Doing so maximizes your chances of building muscle while minimizing your risks for burning out or getting injured.

Chapter 8: Before We End

There's a saying by renowned English playwright John Heywood that though Rome wasn't built in a day, they were busy laying bricks every hour. When it comes to getting your dream physique through calisthenics, it's pretty much the same – you'll need to be patient and cautious.

How can you exercise patience and caution? One is by making sure you're not taking overly ambitious steps. Many people who have dropped out of calisthenics before they were able to get their dream bodies did so because of extreme disappointments, burning out, or getting injured when they tried to shortcut the process by trying to do more than what their bodies were able to handle at the beginning. Their inability to patiently wait for their bodies to adapt to progressively increasing stresses led them to overloading their bodies so much to the point of stopping altogether whether due to discouragements, injuries, or burning out.

Another way to exercise patience and caution is by sticking to proper form when performing the exercises. As much as a dream body is a very worthy goal, it shouldn't be above your overall health and safety. If you give in to the temptation to rush your dream body into existence, you may just prolong it even more when you get injured due to using sloppy form just to eke out more reps and sets.

Lastly, being patient and cautious means giving your body enough time to rest and recover from your workouts. As mentioned earlier, 48 hours is a good guideline for rest and recovery. Don't rush into working out immediately within less than 48 hours from your last calisthenics session. Believe me, your muscles will thank you for it by giving you that body you've always desired – and keep it too – when you respect them enough to give them adequate time to rest and recover.

Conclusion

Calisthenics is definitely one of the best ways to improve agility, become stronger, move faster, build muscle and lose weight. In other words, it's one of the best ways to get your dream body and maintain it. It's because the only equipment you need is yourself, which makes it possible for you to consistently work out anytime and anywhere for free. The only possible hindrance for you in terms of consistently working out with calisthenic exercises is laziness.

But remember, learning the exercises here in this book is just half the battle for your dream body. The other half is action, or applying what you learned. As such, I strongly encourage you to start applying what you learned in this book. In particular, start doing the sample routine and gradually build up your intensity towards your dream body already. The longer you put off action, the higher your risk for non-action becomes, which will prevent you from having that dream body you've always desired.

Here's to your success using calisthenics my friend! Cheers!